Keto Recipes

Snack and

Appetizers

Effective Low-Carb Recipes To Balance Hormones And Effortlessly Reach Your Weight Loss Goal.

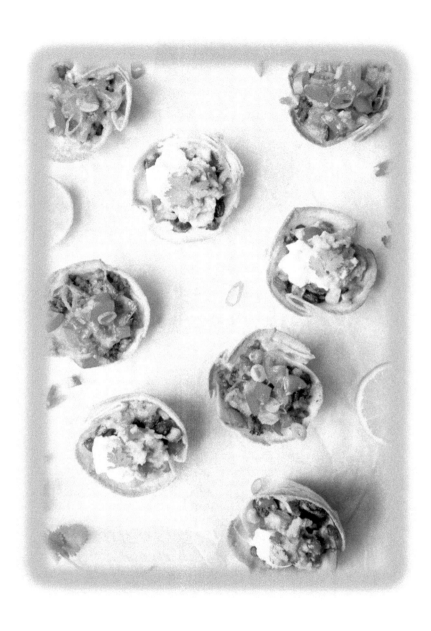

Introduction

Do you want to make a change in your life? Do you want to become a healthier person who can enjoy a new and improved life? Then, you are definitely in the right place. You are about to discover a wonderful and very healthy diet that has changed millions of lives. We are talking about the Ketogenic diet, a lifestyle that will mesmerize you and that will make you a new person in no time.

So, let's sit back, relax and find out more about the Ketogenic diet.

A keto diet is a low carb one. This is the first and one of the most important things you should now. During such a diet, your body makes ketones in your liver and these are used as energy.

Your body will produce less insulin and glucose and a state of ketosis is induced. Ketosis is a natural process that appears when our food intake is lower than usual. The body will soon adapt to this state and therefore you will be able to lose weight in no time but you will also become healthier and your physical and mental performances will improve.

Your blood sugar levels will improve and you won't b predisposed to diabetes. Also, epilepsy and hear diseases can be prevented if you are on a Ketogeni diet.

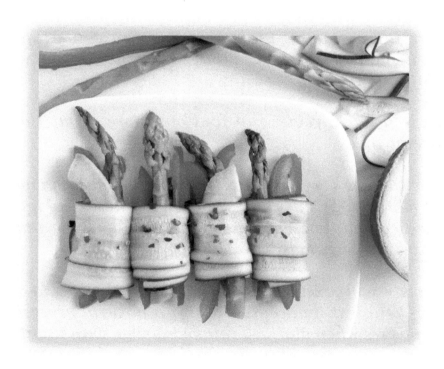

Your cholesterol will improve and you will feel amazing in no time.

How does that sound

A Ketogenic diet is simple and easy to follow as long as you follow some simple rules. You don't need to make huge changes but there are some things you should know.
So, here goes!

Now let's start our magical culinary journey!

Ketogenic lifestyle...here we come!

Enjoy!

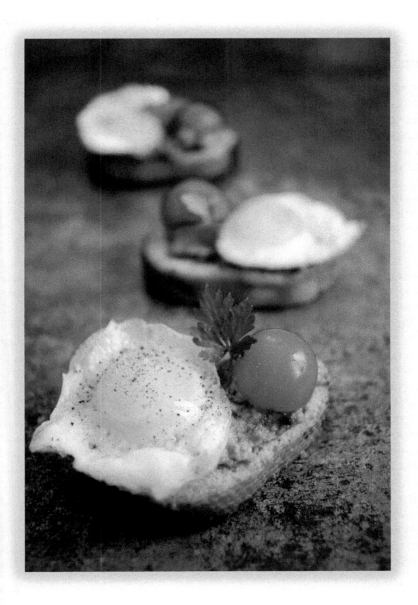

Tasty Zucchini Snack

Try this today!

Preparation time: 10 minutes **Cooking time:** 15 minutes **Servings:** 4

Ingredients:

- 1 cup mozzarella, shredded
- ¼ cup tomato sauce
- 1 zucchini, sliced
- Salt and black pepper to the taste
- A pinch of cumin
- Cooking spray

Directions:

1. Spray a cooking sheet with some oil and arrange zucchini slices.
2. Spread tomato sauce all over zucchini slices, season with salt, pepper and cumin and sprinkle shredded mozzarella.
3. Introduce in the oven at 350 degrees F and bake for 15 minutes.
4. Arrange on a platter and serve.

Enjoy!

Nutrition: calories 140, fat 4, fiber 2, carbs 6, protein 4

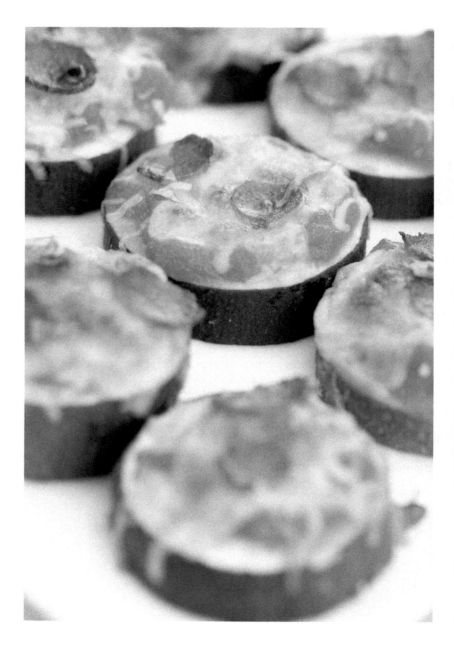

Bacon Delight

Don't be afraid to try this special and very tasty keto snack!

Preparation time: 15 minutes **Cooking time:** 1 hour and 20 minutes **Servings:** 16

Ingredients:

- ½ teaspoon cinnamon, ground
- 2 tablespoons erythritol
- 16 bacon slices
- 1 tablespoon coconut oil
- 3 ounces dark chocolate
- 1 teaspoon maple extract

Directions:

1. In a bowl, mix cinnamon with erythritol and stir.
2. Arrange bacon slices on a lined baking sheet and sprinkle cinnamon mix over them.
3. Flip bacon slices and sprinkle cinnamon mix over them again.
4. Introduce in the oven at 275 degrees F and bake for 1 hour.
5. Heat up a pot with the oil over medium heat, add chocolate and stir until it melts.
6. Add maple extract, stir, take off heat and leave aside to cool down a bit.
7. Take bacon strips out of the oven, leave them to cool down, dip each in chocolate mix, place them on a parchment paper and leave them to cool down completely.
8. Serve cold.

Enjoy!

Nutrition: calories 150, fat 4, fiber 0.4, carbs 1.1, protein 3

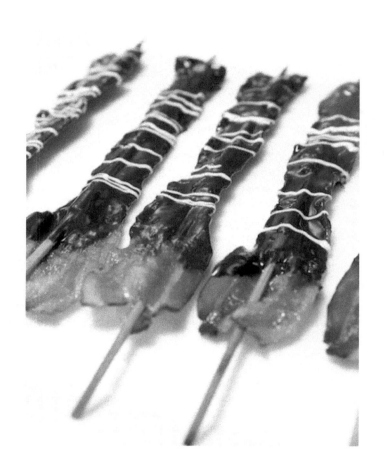

Almond Butter Bars

This is a great keto snack for a casual day!

Preparation time: 2 hours and 10 minutes **Cooking time:** 2 minutes **Servings:** 12

Ingredients:
- ¾ cup coconut, unsweetened and shredded
- ¾ cup almond butter
- ¾ cup stevia
- 1 cup almond butter
- 2 tablespoons almond butter
- 4.5 ounces dark chocolate, chopped
- 2 tablespoons coconut oil

Directions:

1. In a bowl, mix almond flour with stevia and coconut and stir well.
2. Heat up a pan over medium-low heat, add 1 cup almond butter and the coconut oil and whisk well.
3. Add this to almond flour and stir well.
4. Transfer this to a baking dish and press well.
5. Heat up another pan with the chocolate stirring often.
6. Add the rest of the almond butter and whisk well again.
7. Pour this over almond mix and spread evenly.
8. Introduce in the fridge for 2 hours, cut into 12 bars and serve as a keto snack.

Enjoy!

Nutrition: calories 140, fat 2, fiber 1, carbs 5, protein 1

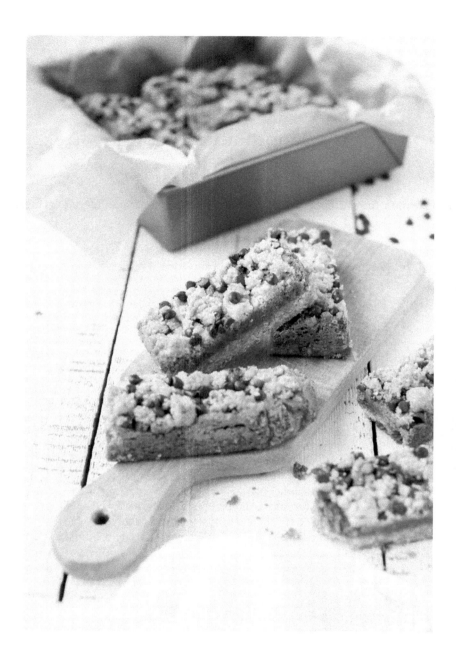

Zucchini Chips

Enjoy a great snack with only a few calories!

Preparation time: 10 minutes **Cooking time:** 3 hours **Servings:** 8

Ingredients:

- 3 zucchinis, very thinly sliced
- Salt and black pepper to the taste
- 2 tablespoons olive oil
- 2 tablespoons balsamic vinegar

Directions:

1. In a bowl, mix oil with vinegar, salt and pepper and whisk well.
2. Add zucchini slices, toss to coat well and spread on a lined baking sheet, introduce in the oven at 200 degrees F and bake for 3 hours.
3. Leave chips to cool down and serve them as a keto snack.

Enjoy!

Nutrition: calories 40, fat 3, fiber 7, carbs 3, protein 7

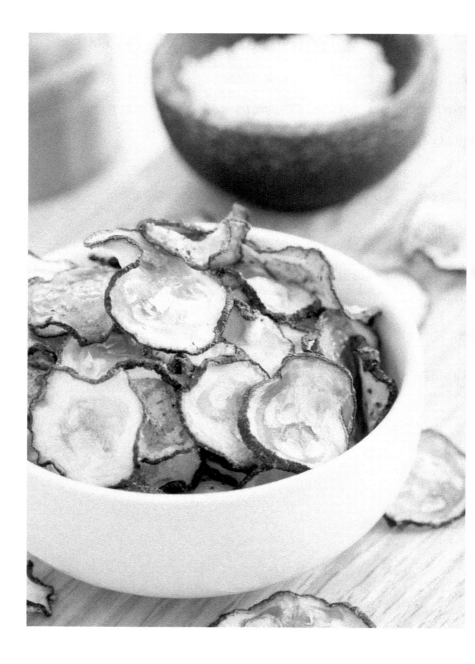

Simple Hummus

Everyone loves a good hummus! Try this one!

Preparation time: 10 minutes **Cooking time:** 0 minutes **Servings:** 5

Ingredients:
- 4 cups zucchinis, finely chopped
- ¼ cup olive oil
- Salt and black pepper to the taste
- 4 garlic cloves, minced
- ¾ cup tahini
- ½ cup lemon juice
- 1 tablespoon cumin, ground

Directions:
1. In your blender, mix zucchinis with salt, pepper, oil, lemon juice, garlic, tahini and cumin and blend very well.
2. Transfer to a bowl and serve.

Enjoy!

Nutrition: calories 80, fat 5, fiber 3, carbs 6, protein 7

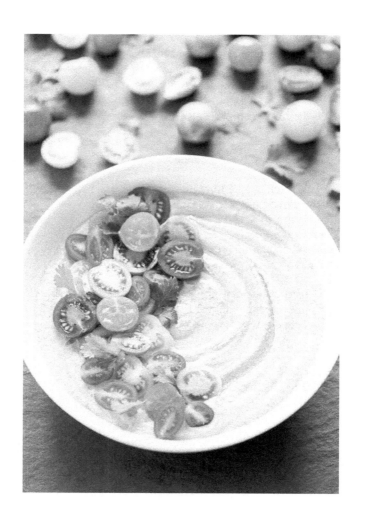

Amazing Celery Sticks

This is so great! It's an amazing keto snack, indeed!

Preparation time: 10 minutes **Cooking time:** 0 minutes **Servings:** 12

Ingredients:

- 2 cups rotisserie chicken, shredded
- 6 celery sticks cut in halves
- 3 tablespoons hot tomato sauce
- ¼ cup mayonnaise
- Salt and black pepper to the taste
- ½ teaspoon garlic powder
- Some chopped chives for serving

Directions:

1. In a bowl, mix chicken with salt, pepper, garlic powder, mayo and tomato sauce and stir well.
2. Arrange celery pieces on a platter, spread chicken mix over them, sprinkle some chives and serve.

Enjoy!

Nutrition: calories 100, fat 2, fiber 3, carbs 1, protein 6

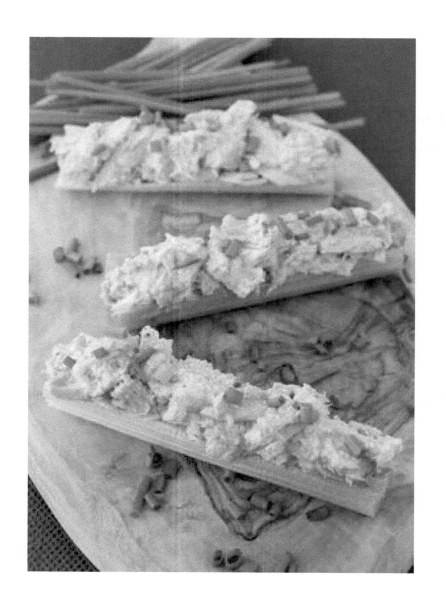

Beef Jerky Snack

We are sure you will love this keto snack!

Preparation time: 6 hours **Cooking time:** 4 hours **Servings:** 6

Ingredients:
- 24 ounces amber
- 2 cups soy sauce
- ½ cup Worcestershire sauce
- 2 tablespoons black peppercorns
- 2 tablespoons black pepper
- 2 pounds beef round, sliced

Directions:

1. In a bowl, mix soy sauce with black peppercorns, black pepper and Worcestershire sauce and whisk well.
2. Add beef slices, toss to coat and leave aside in the fridge for 6 hours.
3. Spread this on a rack, introduce in the oven at 370 degrees F and bake for 4 hours.
4. Transfer to a bowl and serve.

Enjoy!

Nutrition: calories 300, fat 12, fiber 4, carbs 3, protein 8

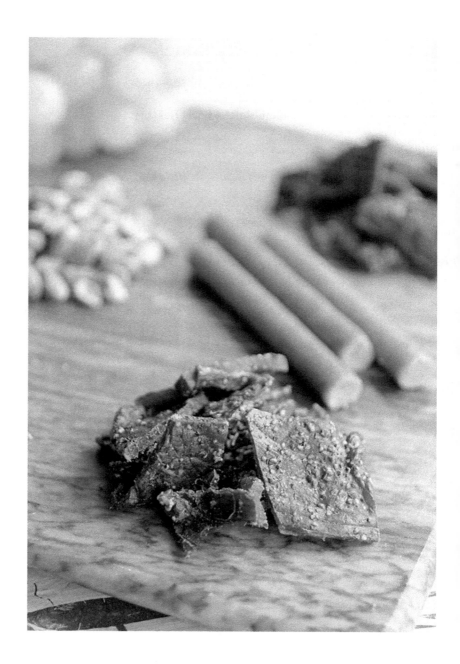

Crab Dip

You will adore this amazing keto appetizer!

Preparation time: 10 minutes **Cooking time:** 30 minutes **Servings:** 8

Ingredients:

- 8 bacon strips, sliced
- 12 ounces crab meat
- ½ cup mayonnaise
- ½ cup sour cream
- 8 ounces cream cheese
- 2 poblano pepper, chopped
- 2 tablespoons lemon juice
- Salt and black pepper to the taste
- 4 garlic cloves, minced
- 4 green onions, minced
- ½ cup parmesan cheese+ ½ cup parmesan cheese, grated
- Salt and black pepper to the taste

Directions:

1. Heat up a pan over medium high heat, add bacon, cook until it's crispy, transfer to paper towels, chop and leave aside to cool down.
2. In a bowl, mix sour cream with cream cheese and mayo and stir well.
3. Add ½ cup parmesan, poblano peppers, bacon, green onion, garlic and lemon juice and stir again.
4. Add crab meat, salt and pepper and stir gently.
5. Pour this into a heatproof baking dish, spread the rest of the parm, introduce in the oven and bake at 350 degrees F for 20 minutes.
6. Serve your dip warm with cucumber stick.

Enjoy!

Nutrition: calories 200, fat 7, fiber 2, carbs 4, protein 6

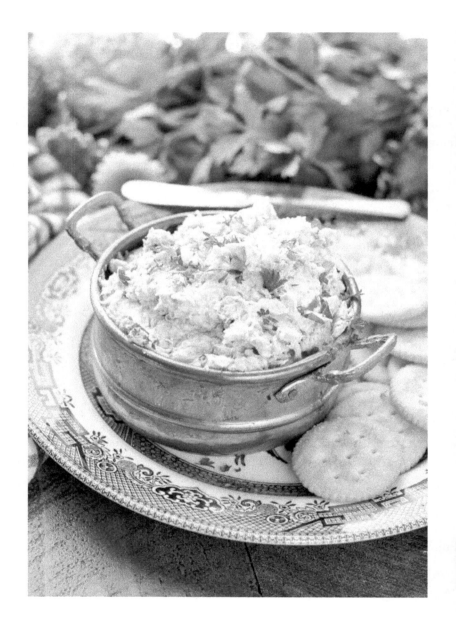

Simple Spinach Balls

This is a very tasty keto party appetizer!

Preparation time: 10 minutes **Cooking time:** 12 minutes **Servings:** 30

Ingredients:
- 4 tablespoons melted ghee
- 2 eggs
- 1 cup almond flour
- 16 ounces spinach
- 1/3 cup feta cheese, crumbled
- ¼ teaspoon nutmeg, ground
- 1/3 cup parmesan, grated
- Salt and black pepper to the taste
- 1 tablespoon onion powder
- 3 tablespoons whipping cream
- 1 teaspoon garlic powder

Directions:
1. In your blender, mix spinach with ghee, eggs, almond flour, feta cheese, parmesan, nutmeg, whipping cream, salt, pepper, onion and garlic pepper and blend very well.
2. Transfer to a bowl and keep in the freezer for 10 minutes
3. Shape 30 spinach balls, arrange on a lined baking sheet, introduce in the oven at 350 degrees F and bake for 12 minutes.
4. Leave spinach balls to cool down and serve as a party appetizer.

Enjoy!

Nutrition: calories 60, fat 5, fiber 1, carbs 0.7, protein 2

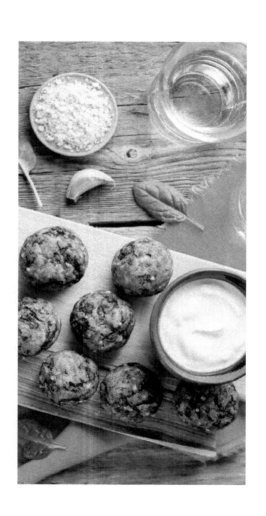

Tasty Pepper Nachos

These look wonderful! They are so tasty and healthy!

Preparation time: 10 minutes **Cooking time:** 20 minutes **Servings:** 6

Ingredients:

- 1 pound mini bell peppers, cut in halves
- Salt and black pepper to the taste
- 1 teaspoon garlic powder
- 1 teaspoon sweet paprika
- ½ teaspoon oregano, dried
- ¼ teaspoon red pepper flakes
- 1 pound beef meat, ground
- 1 and ½ cups cheddar cheese, shredded
- 1 tablespoons chili powder
- 1 teaspoon cumin, ground
- ½ cup tomato, chopped
- Sour cream for serving

Directions:

1. In a bowl, mix chili powder with paprika, salt, pepper, cumin, oregano, pepper flakes and garlic powder and stir.
2. Heat up a pan over medium heat, add beef, stir and brown for 10 minutes.
3. Add chili powder mix, stir and take off heat.
4. Arrange pepper halves on a lined baking sheet, stuff them with the beef mix, sprinkle cheese, introduce in the oven at 400 degrees F and bake for 10 minutes.
5. Take peppers out of the oven, sprinkle tomatoes and divide between plates and serve with sour cream on top.

Enjoy!

Nutrition: calories 350, fat 22, fiber 3, carbs 6, protein 27

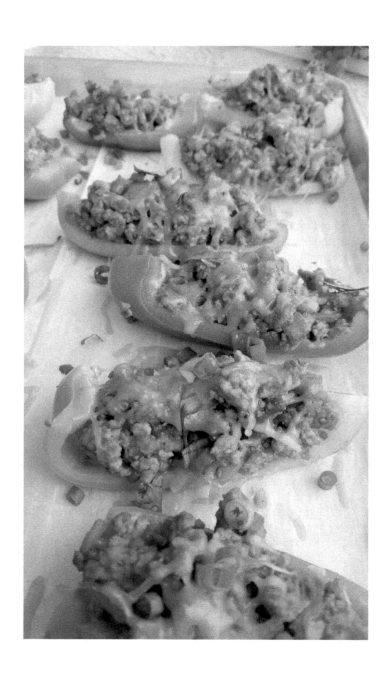

Garlic Spinach Dip

This keto appetizer will make you love spinach even more!

Preparation time: 10 minutes **Cooking time:** 35 minutes **Servings:** 6

ngredients:

- 6 bacon slices
- 5 ounces spinach
- ½ cup sour cream
- 8 ounces cream cheese, soft
- 1 and ½ tablespoons parsley, chopped
- 2.5 ounces parmesan, grated
- 1 tablespoon lemon juice
- Salt and black pepper to the taste
- 1 tablespoon garlic, minced

Directions:

1. Heat up a pan over medium heat, add bacon, cook until it's crispy, transfer to paper towels, drain grease, crumble and leave aside in a bowl.
2. Heat up the same pan with the bacon grease over medium heat, add spinach, stir, cook for 2 minutes and transfer to a bowl.
3. In another bowl, mix cream cheese with garlic, salt, pepper, sour cream and parsley and stir well.
4. Add bacon and stir again.
5. Add lemon juice and spinach and stir everything.
6. Add parmesan and stir again.
7. Divide this into ramekins, introduce in the oven at 350 degrees f and bake for 25 minutes.
8. Turn oven to broil and broil for 4 minutes more.
9. Serve with crackers.

Enjoy!

Nutrition: calories 345, fat 12, fiber 3, carbs 6, protein 11

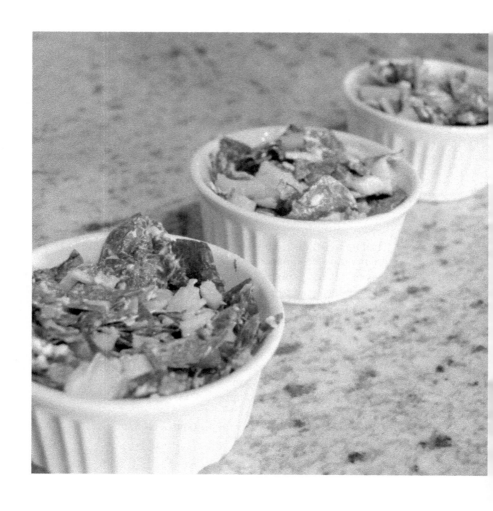

Mushrooms Appetizer

These mushrooms are so yummy!

Preparation time: 10 minutes **Cooking time:** 20 minutes **Servings:** 5

Ingredients:
- ¼ cup mayo
- 1 teaspoon garlic powder
- 1 small yellow onion, chopped
- 24 ounces white mushroom caps
- Salt and black pepper to the taste
- 1 teaspoon curry powder
- 4 ounces cream cheese, soft
- ¼ cup sour cream
- ½ cup Mexican cheese, shredded
- 1 cup shrimp, cooked, peeled, deveined and chopped

Directions:
1. In a bowl, mix mayo with garlic powder, onion, curry powder, cream cheese, sour cream, Mexican cheese, shrimp, salt and pepper to the taste and whisk well.
2. Stuff mushrooms with this mix, place on a baking sheet and cook in the oven at 350 degrees F for 20 minutes.
3. Arrange on a platter and serve.

Enjoy!

Nutrition: calories 244, fat 20, fiber 3, carbs 7, protein 14

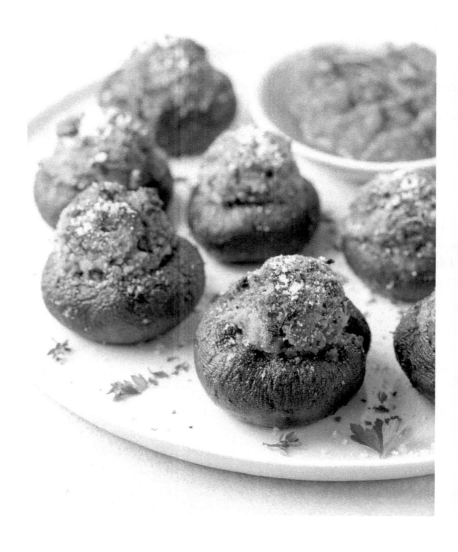

Simple Bread Sticks

You just have to give this amazing keto snack a chance!

Preparation time: 10 minutes **Cooking time:** 15 minutes **Servings:** 24

Ingredients:

- 3 tablespoons cream cheese, soft
- 1 tablespoon psyllium powder
- ¾ cup almond flour
- 2 cups mozzarella cheese, melted for 30 seconds in the microwave
- 1 teaspoon baking powder
- 1 egg
- 2 tablespoons Italian seasoning
- Salt and black pepper to the taste
- 3 ounces cheddar cheese, grated
- 1 teaspoon onion powder

Directions:

1. In a bowl, mix psyllium powder with almond flour, baking powder, salt and pepper and whisk.
2. Add cream cheese, melted mozzarella and egg and stir using your hands until you obtain a dough.
3. Spread this on a baking sheet and cut into 24 sticks.
4. Sprinkle onion powder and Italian seasoning over them.
5. Top with cheddar cheese, introduce in the oven at 350 degrees F and bake for 15 minutes.
6. Serve them as a keto snack!

Enjoy!

Nutrition: calories 245, fat 12, fiber 5, carbs 3, protein 14

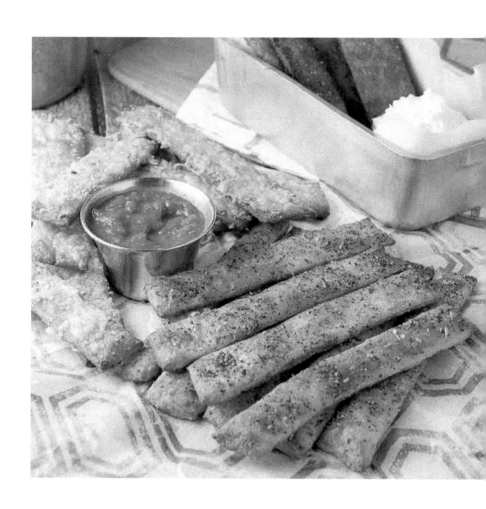

Italian Meatballs

This Italian-style appetizer is 100% keto!

Preparation time: 10 minutes **Cooking time:** 6 minutes **Servings:** 16

Ingredients:

- 1 egg
- Salt and black pepper to the taste
- ¼ cup almond flour
- 1 pound turkey meat, ground
- ½ teaspoon garlic powder
- 2 tablespoons sun-dried tomatoes, chopped
- ½ cup mozzarella cheese, shredded
- 2 tablespoons olive oil
- 2 tablespoon basil, chopped

Directions:

1. In a bowl, mix turkey with salt, pepper, egg, almond flour, garlic powder, sun-dried tomatoes, mozzarella and basil and stir well.
2. Shape 12 meatballs, heat up a pan with the oil over medium high heat, drop meatballs and cook them for 2 minutes on each side.
3. Arrange on a platter and serve.

Enjoy!

Nutrition: calories 80, fat 6, fiber 3, carbs 5, protein 7

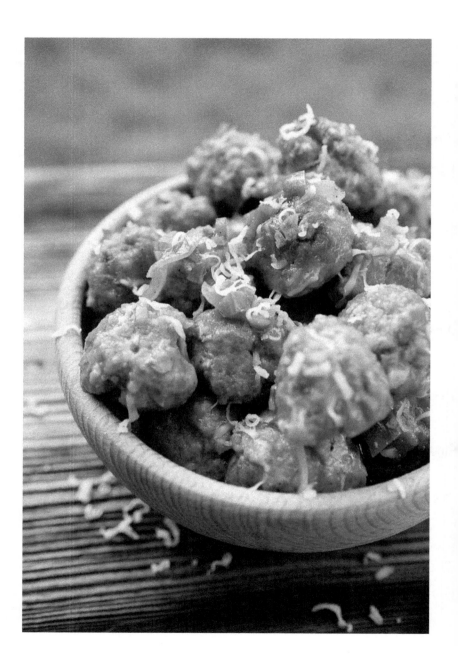

Parmesan Wings

These will be appreciated by all your family!

Preparation time: 10 minutes **Cooking time:** 24 minutes **Servings:** 6

Ingredients:
- 6-pound chicken wings, cut in halves
- Salt and black pepper to the taste
- ½ teaspoon Italian seasoning
- 2 tablespoons ghee
- ½ cup parmesan cheese, grated
- A pinch of red pepper flakes, crushed
- 1 teaspoon garlic powder
- 1 egg

Directions:
1. Arrange chicken wings on a lined baking sheet, introduce in the oven at 425 degrees F and bake for 17 minutes.
2. Meanwhile, in your blender, mix ghee with cheese, egg, salt, pepper, pepper flakes, garlic powder and Italian seasoning and blend very well.
3. Take chicken wings out of the oven, flip them, turn oven to broil and broil them for 5 minutes more.
4. Take chicken pieces out of the oven again, pour sauce over them, toss to coat well and broil for 1 minute more.
5. Serve them as a quick keto appetizer.

Enjoy!

Nutrition: calories 134, fat 8, fiber 1, carbs 0.5, protein 14

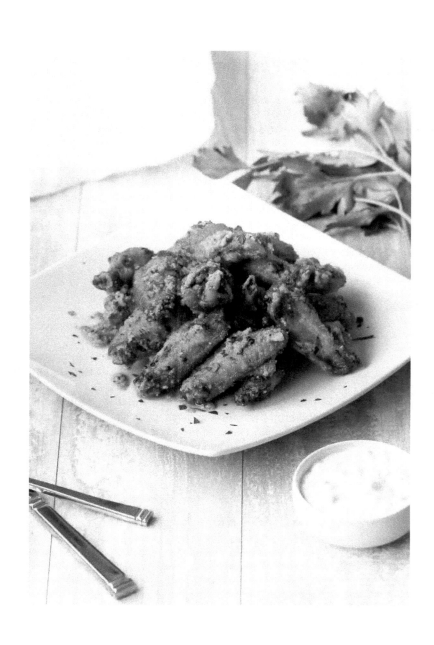

Cheese Sticks

This keto appetizer will simply melt into your mouth!

Preparation time: 1 hour and 10 minutes **Cooking time:** 20 minutes **Servings:** 16

Ingredients:
- 2 eggs, whisked
- Salt and black pepper to the taste
- 8 mozzarella cheese strings, cut in halves
- 1 cup parmesan, grated
- 1 tablespoon Italian seasoning
- ½ cup olive oil
- 1 garlic clove, minced

Directions:

1. In a bowl, mix parmesan with salt, pepper, Italian seasoning and garlic and stir well.
2. Put whisked eggs in another bowl.
3. Dip mozzarella sticks in egg mixture, then in the cheese mix.
4. Dip them again in egg and in parm mix and keep them in the freezer for 1 hour.
5. Heat up a pan with the oil over medium high heat, add cheese sticks, fry them until they are golden on one side, flip and cook them the same way on the other side.
6. Arrange them on a platter and serve.

Enjoy!

Nutrition: calories 140, fat 5, fiber 1, carbs 3, protein 4

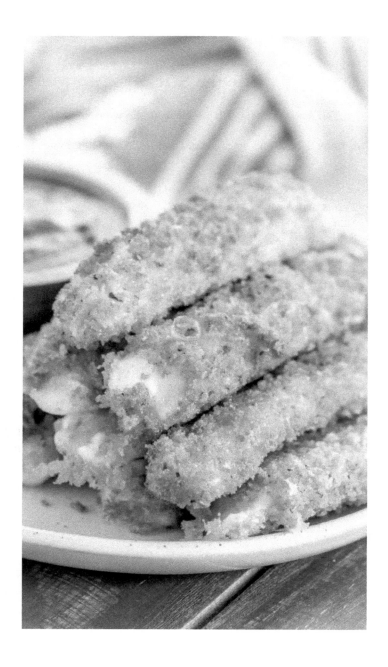

Tasty Broccoli Sticks

You must invite all your friends to taste this keto appetizer!

Preparation time: 10 minutes **Cooking time:** 20 minutes **Servings:** 20

Ingredients:
- 1 egg
- 2 cups broccoli florets
- 1/3 cup cheddar cheese, grated
- ¼ cup yellow onion, chopped
- 1/3 cup panko breadcrumbs
- 1/3 cup Italian breadcrumbs
- 2 tablespoons parsley, chopped
- A drizzle of olive oil
- Salt and black pepper to the taste

Directions:
1. Heat up a pot with water over medium heat, add broccoli, steam for 1 minute, drain, chop and put into a bowl.
2. Add egg, cheddar cheese, panko and Italian bread crumbs, salt, pepper and parsley and stir everything well.
3. Shape sticks out of this mix using your hands and place them on a baking sheet which you've greased with some olive oil.
4. Introduce in the oven at 400 degrees F and bake for 20 minutes.
5. Arrange on a platter and serve.

Enjoy!

Nutrition: calories 100, fat 4, fiber 2, carbs 7, protein 7

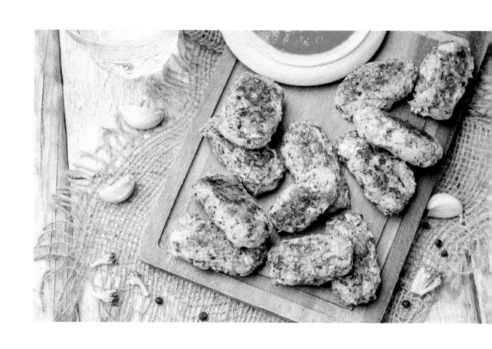

Taco Cups

These taco cups make the perfect party appetizer!

Preparation time: 10 minutes **Cooking time:** 40 minutes **Servings:** 30

Ingredients:
- 1 pound beef, ground
- 2 cups cheddar cheese, shredded
- ¼ cup water
- Salt and black pepper to the taste
- 2 tablespoons cumin
- 2 tablespoons chili powder
- Pico de gallo for serving

Directions:

1. Divide spoonful of parmesan on a lined baking sheet, introduce in the oven at 350 degrees F and bake for 7 minutes.
2. Leave cheese to cool down for 1 minute, transfer them to mini cupcake molds and shape them into cups.
3. Meanwhile, heat up a pan over medium high heat, add beef, stir and cook until it browns.
4. Add the water, salt, pepper, cumin and chili powder, stir and cook for 5 minutes more.
5. Divide into cheese cups, top with pico de gallo, transfer them all to a platter and serve.

Enjoy!

Nutrition: calories 140, fat 6, fiber 0, carbs 6, protein 15

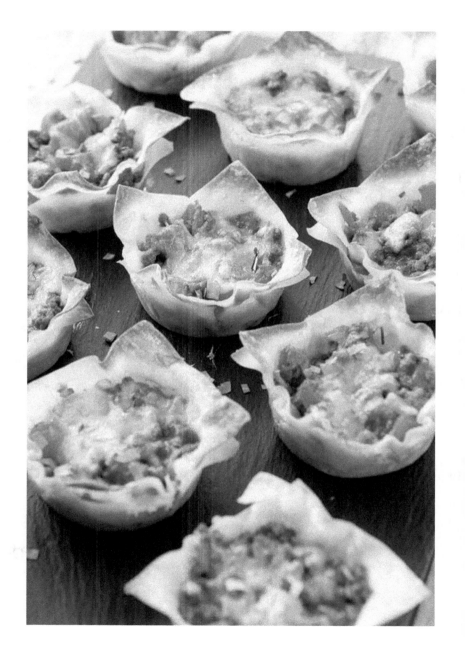

Tasty Chicken Egg Rolls

These are just what you need! It's the best keto party appetizer!

Preparation time: 2 hours and 10 minutes **Cooking time:** 15 minutes **Servings:** 12

Ingredients:
- 4 ounces blue cheese
- 2 cups chicken, cooked and finely chopped
- Salt and black pepper to the taste
- 2 green onions, chopped
- 2 celery stalks, finely chopped
- ½ cup tomato sauce
- ½ teaspoon erythritol
- 12 egg roll wrappers
- Vegetable oil

Directions:
1. In a bowl, mix chicken meat with blue cheese, salt, pepper, green onions, celery, tomato sauce and sweetener, stir well and keep in the fridge for 2 hours.
2. Place egg wrappers on a working surface, divide chicken mix on them, roll and seal edges.
3. Heat up a pan with vegetable oil over medium high heat, add egg rolls, cook until they are golden, flip and cook on the other side as well.
4. Arrange on a platter and serve them.

Enjoy!

Nutrition: calories 220, fat 7, fiber 2, carbs 6, protein 10

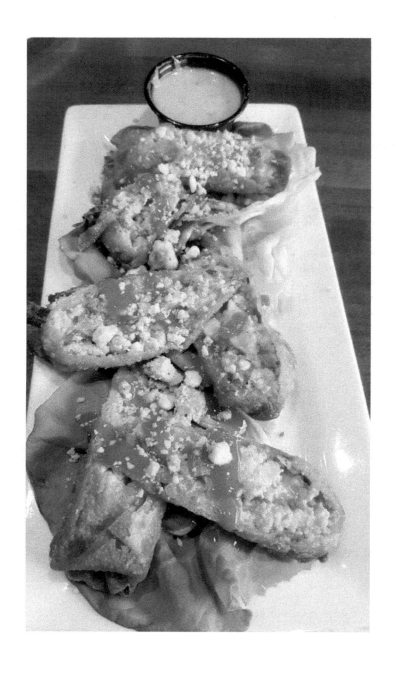

Halloumi Cheese Fries

These are so crunchy and delightful!

Preparation time: 10 minutes **Cooking time:** 5 minutes **Servings:** 4

ngredients:
- 1 cup marinara sauce
- 8 ounces halloumi cheese, pat dried and sliced into fries
- 2 ounces tallow

Directions:

1. Heat up a pan with the tallow over medium high heat.
2. Add halloumi pieces, cover, cook for 2 minutes on each side and transfer to paper towels.
3. Drain excess grease, transfer them to a bowl and serve with marinara sauce on the side.

Enjoy!

Nutrition: calories 200, fat 16, fiber 1, carbs 1, protein 13

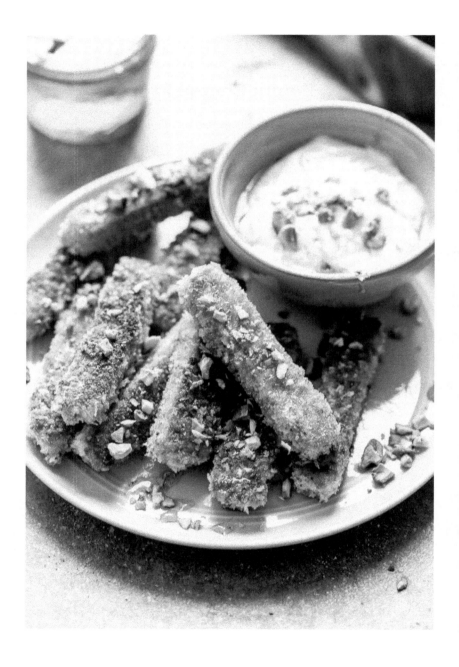

Jalapeno Crisps

These are so easy to make at home!

Preparation time: 10 minutes **Cooking time:** 25 minutes **Servings:** 20

Ingredients:
- 3 tablespoons olive oil
- 5 jalapenos, sliced
- 8 ounces parmesan cheese, grated
- ½ teaspoon onion powder
- Salt and black pepper to the taste
- Tabasco sauce for serving

Directions:

1. In a bowl, mix jalapeno slices with salt, pepper, oil and onion powder, toss to coat and spread on a lined baking sheet.
2. Introduce in the oven at 450 degrees F and bake for 15 minutes.
3. Take jalapeno slices out of the oven, leave them to cool down.
4. In a bowl, mix pepper slices with the cheese and press well.
5. Arrange all slices on an another lined baking sheet, introduce in the oven again and bake for 10 minutes more.
6. Leave jalapenos to cool down, arrange on a plate and serve with Tabasco sauce on the side.

Enjoy!

Nutrition: calories 50, fat 3, fiber 0.1, carbs 0.3, protein 2

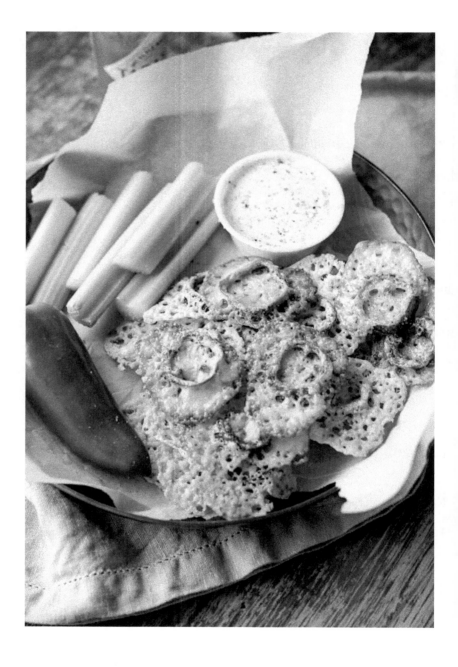

Delicious Cucumber Cups

Get ready to taste something really elegant and delicious!

Preparation time: 10 minutes **Cooking time:** 0 minutes **Servings:** 24

Ingredients:

- 2 cucumbers, peeled, cut into ¾ inch slices and some of the seeds scooped out
- ½ cup sour cream
- Salt and white pepper to the taste
- 6 ounces smoked salmon, flaked
- 1/3 cup cilantro, chopped
- 2 teaspoons lime juice
- 1 tablespoon lime zest
- A pinch of cayenne pepper

Directions:

1. In a bowl mix salmon with salt, pepper, cayenne, sour cream, lime juice and zest and cilantro and stir well.
2. Fill each cucumber cup with this salmon mix, arrange on a platter and serve as a keto appetizer.

Enjoy!

Nutrition: calories 30, fat 11, fiber 1, carbs 1, protein 2

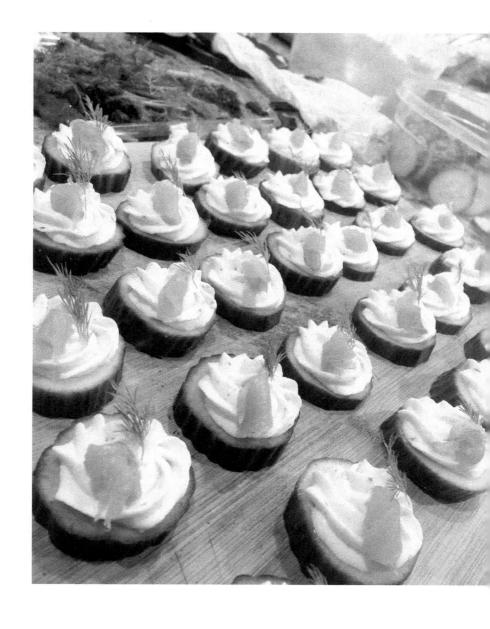

Caviar Salad

This is so elegant! It's so delicious and sophisticated!

Preparation time: 6 minutes **Cooking time:** 0 minutes **Servings:** 16

Ingredients:
- 8 eggs, hard-boiled, peeled and mashed with a fork
- 4 ounces black caviar
- 4 ounces red caviar
- Salt and black pepper to the taste
- 1 yellow onion, finely chopped
- ¾ cup mayonnaise
- Some toast baguette slices for serving

Directions:

1. In a bowl, mix mashed eggs with mayo, salt, pepper and onion and stir well.
2. Spread eggs salad on toasted baguette slices, and top each with caviar.

Enjoy!

Nutrition: calories 122, fat 8, fiber 1, carbs 4, protein 7

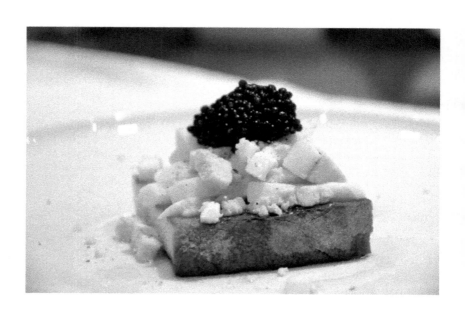

Marinated Kebabs

This is the perfect appetizer for a summer barbecue!

Preparation time: 20 minutes **Cooking time:** 10 minutes **Servings:** 6

Ingredients:
- 1 red bell pepper, cut into chunks
- 1 green bell pepper, cut into chunks
- 1 orange bell pepper, cut into chunks
- 2 pounds sirloin steak, cut into medium cubes
- 4 garlic cloves, minced
- 1 red onion, cut into chunks
- Salt and black pepper to the taste
- 2 tablespoons Dijon mustard
- 2 and ½ tablespoons Worcestershire sauce
- ¼ cup tamari sauce
- ¼ cup lemon juice
- ½ cup olive oil

Directions:
1. In a bowl, mix Worcestershire sauce with salt, pepper, garlic, mustard, tamari, lemon juice and oil and whisk very well.
2. Add beef, bell peppers and onion chunks to this mix, toss to coat and leave aside for a few minutes.
3. Arrange bell pepper, meat cubes and onion chunks on skewers alternating colors, place them on your preheated grill over medium high heat, cook for 5 minutes on each side, transfer to a platter and serve as a summer keto appetizer.

Enjoy!

Nutrition: calories 246, fat 12, fiber 1, carbs 4, protein 26

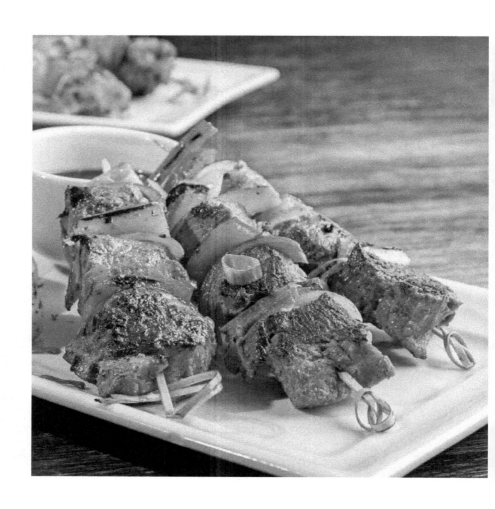

Simple Zucchini Rolls

You've got to try this simple and very tasty appetizer as soon as possible!

Preparation time: 10 minutes **Cooking time:** 5 minutes **Servings:** 24

Ingredients:
- 2 tablespoons olive oil
- 3 zucchinis, thinly sliced
- 24 basil leaves
- 2 tablespoons mint, chopped
- 1 and 1/3 cup ricotta cheese
- Salt and black pepper to the taste
- ¼ cup basil, chopped
- Tomato sauce for serving

Directions:
1. Brush zucchini slices with the olive oil, season with salt and pepper on both sides, place them on preheated grill over medium heat, cook them for 2 minutes, flip and cook for another 2 minutes.
2. Place zucchini slices on a plate and leave aside for now.
3. In a bowl, mix ricotta with chopped basil, mint, salt and pepper and stir well.
4. Spread this over zucchini slices, divide whole basil leaves as well, roll and serve as an appetizer with some tomato sauce on the side.

Enjoy!

Nutrition: calories 40, fat 3, fiber 0.3, carbs 1, protein 2

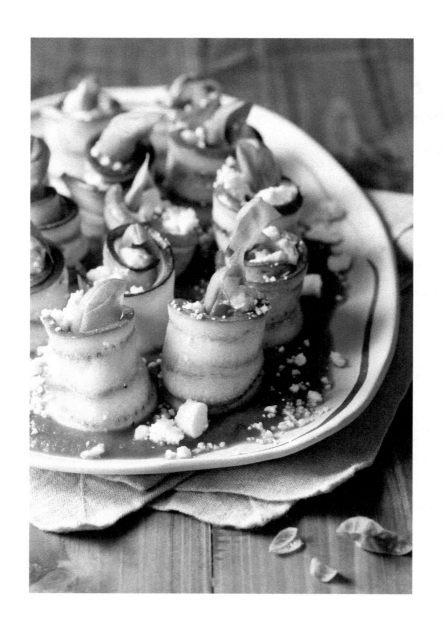

Simple Green Crackers

These are real fun to make and they taste amazing!

Preparation time: 10 minutes **Cooking time:** 24 hours **Servings:** 6

Ingredients:
- 2 cups flax seed, ground
- 2 cups flax seed, soaked overnight and drained
- 4 bunches kale, chopped
- 1 bunch basil, chopped
- ½ bunch celery, chopped
- 4 garlic cloves, minced
- 1/3 cup olive oil

Directions:

1. In your food processor mix ground flaxseed with celery, kale, basil and garlic and blend well.
2. Add oil and soaked flaxseed and blend again.
3. Spread this on a tray, cut into medium crackers, introduce in your dehydrator and dry for 24 hours at 115 degrees F, turning them halfway.
4. Arrange them on a platter and serve.

Enjoy!

Nutrition: calories 100, fat 1, fiber 2, carbs 1, protein 4

ì

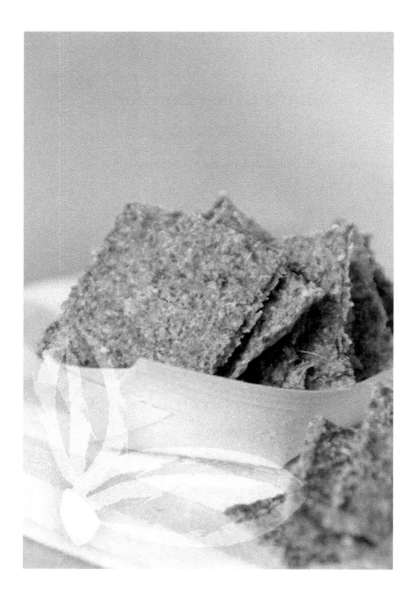

Cheese And Pesto Terrine

This looks so amazing and it tastes great!

Preparation time: 30 minutes **Cooking time:** 0 minutes **Servings:** 10

Ingredients:
- ½ cup heavy cream
- 10 ounces goat cheese, crumbled
- 3 tablespoons basil pesto
- Salt and black pepper to the taste
- 5 sun-dried tomatoes, chopped
- ¼ cup pine nuts, toasted and chopped
- 1 tablespoons pine nuts, toasted and chopped

Directions:

1. In a bowl, mix goat cheese with the heavy cream, salt and pepper and stir using your mixer.
2. Spoon half of this mix into a lined bowl and spread.
3. Add pesto on top and also spread.
4. Add another layer of cheese, then add sun dried tomatoes and ¼ cup pine nuts.
5. Spread one last layer of cheese and top with 1 tablespoon pine nuts.
6. Keep in the fridge for a while, turn upside down on a plate and serve.

Enjoy!

Nutrition: calories 240, fat 12, fiber 3, carbs 5, protein 12

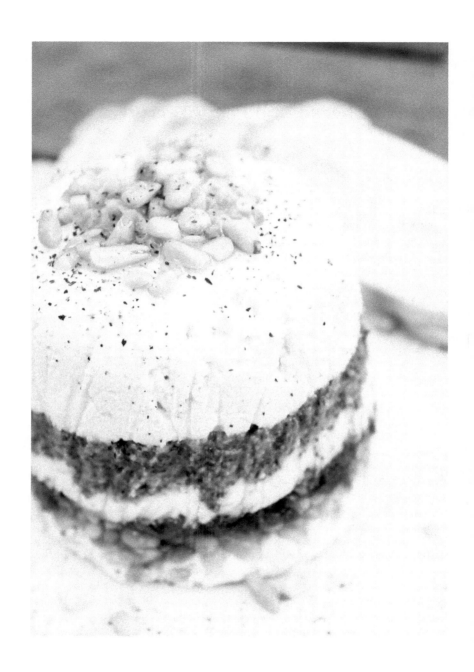

Avocado Salsa

You will make this over and over again! That's how tasty it is!

Preparation time: 10 minutes **Cooking time:** 0 minutes **Servings:** 4

Ingredients:
- 1 small red onion, chopped
- 2 avocados, pitted, peeled and chopped
- 3 jalapeno pepper, chopped
- Salt and black pepper to the taste
- 2 tablespoons cumin powder
- 2 tablespoons lime juice
- ½ tomato, chopped

Directions:

1. In a bowl, mix onion with avocados, peppers, salt, black pepper, cumin, lime juice and tomato pieces and stir well.
2. Transfer this to a bowl and serve with toasted baguette slices as a keto appetizer.

Enjoy!

Nutrition: calories 120, fat 2, fiber 2, carbs 0.4, protein 4

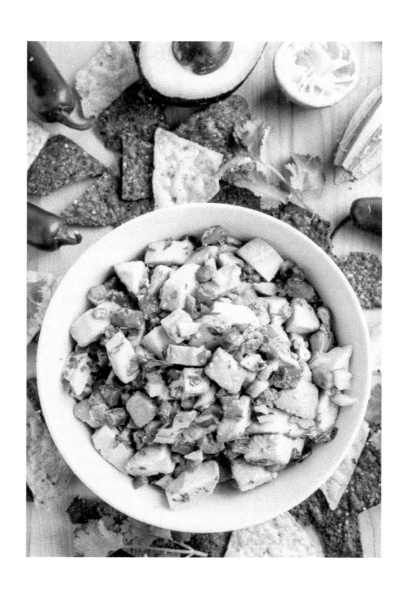

Tasty Egg Chips

Do you want to impress everyone? Then, try these chips!

Preparation time: 5 minutes **Cooking time:** 10 minutes **Servings:** 2

Ingredients:
- ½ tablespoon water
- 2 tablespoons parmesan, shredded
- 4 eggs whites
- Salt and black pepper to the taste

Directions:
1. In a bowl, mix egg whites with salt, pepper and water and whisk well.
2. Spoon this into a muffin pan, sprinkle cheese on top, introduce in the oven at 400 degrees F and bake for 15 minutes.
3. Transfer egg white chips to a platter and serve with a keto dip on the side.

Enjoy!

Nutrition: calories 120, fat 2, fiber 1, carbs 2, protein 7

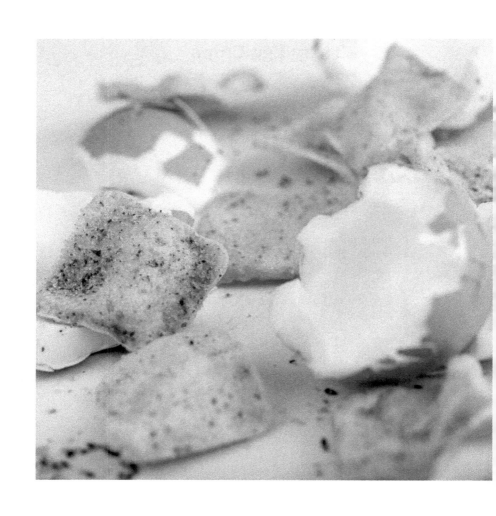

Chili Lime Chips

These crackers will impress you with their amazing taste!

Preparation time: 10 minutes **Cooking time:** 20 minutes **Servings:** 4

Ingredients:
- 1 cup almond flour
- Salt and black pepper to the taste
- 1 and ½ teaspoons lime zest
- 1 teaspoon lime juice
- 1 egg

Directions:

1. In a bowl, mix almond flour with lime zest, lime juice and salt and stir.
2. Add egg and whisk well again.
3. Divide this into 4 parts, roll each into a ball and then spread well using a rolling pin.
4. Cut each into 6 triangles, place them all on a lined baking sheet, introduce in the oven at 350 degrees F and bake for 20 minutes.

Enjoy!

Nutrition: calories 90, fat 1, fiber 1, carbs 0.6, protein 3

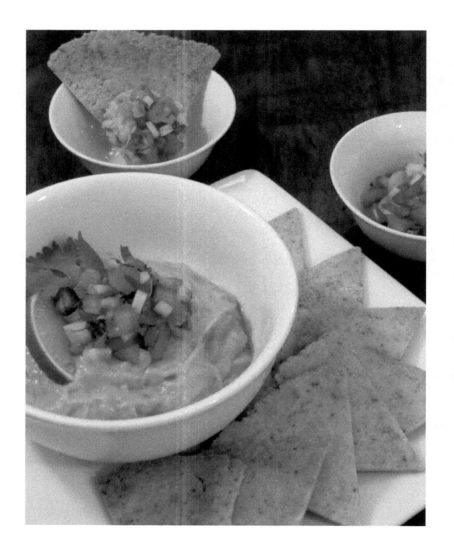

Artichoke Dip

It's so rich and flavored!

Preparation time: 10 minutes **Cooking time:** 15 minutes **Servings:** 16

Ingredients:

- ¼ cup sour cream
- ¼ cup heavy cream
- ¼ cup mayonnaise
- ¼ cup shallot, chopped
- 1 tablespoon olive oil
- 2 garlic cloves, minced
- 4 ounces cream cheese
- ½ cup parmesan cheese, grated
- 1 cup mozzarella cheese, shredded
- 4 ounces feta cheese, crumbled
- 1 tablespoon balsamic vinegar
- 28 ounces canned artichoke hearts, chopped
- Salt and black pepper to the taste
- 10 ounces spinach, chopped

Directions:

1. Heat up a pan with the oil over medium heat, add shallot and garlic, stir and cook for 3 minutes.
2. Add heavy cream and cream cheese and stir.
3. Also add sour cream, parmesan, mayo, feta cheese and mozzarella cheese, stir and reduce heat.
4. Add artichoke, spinach, salt, pepper and vinegar, stir well, take off heat and transfer to a bowl.
5. Serve as a tasty keto dip.

Enjoy!

Nutrition: calories 144, fat 12, fiber 2, carbs 5, protein 5

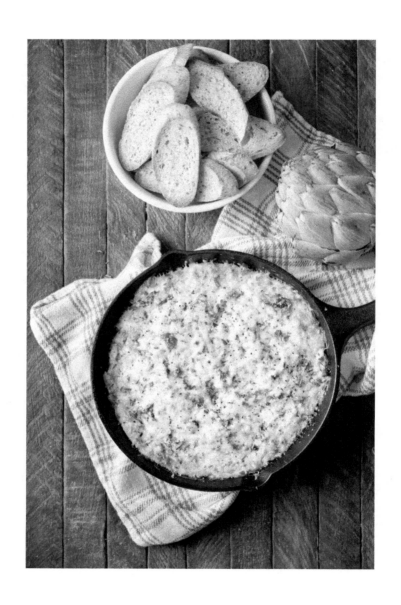

Conclusion

This is really a life changing cookbook. It shows you everything you need to know about the Ketogenic diet and it helps you get started.

You now know some of the best and most popular Ketogenic recipes in the world.

We have something for everyone's taste!

So, don't hesitate too much and start your new life as a follower of the Ketogenic diet!

Get your hands on this special recipes collection and start cooking in this new, exciting and healthy way!

Have a lot of fun and enjoy your Ketogenic diet!

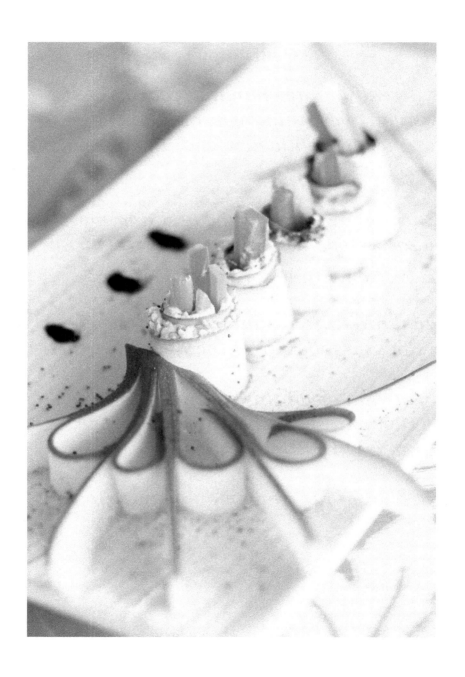

Lightning Source UK Ltd.
Milton Keynes UK
UKHW020643270521
384471UK00010B/722